A Handy Guide to
Essential

YOGA

Poses & Sequences

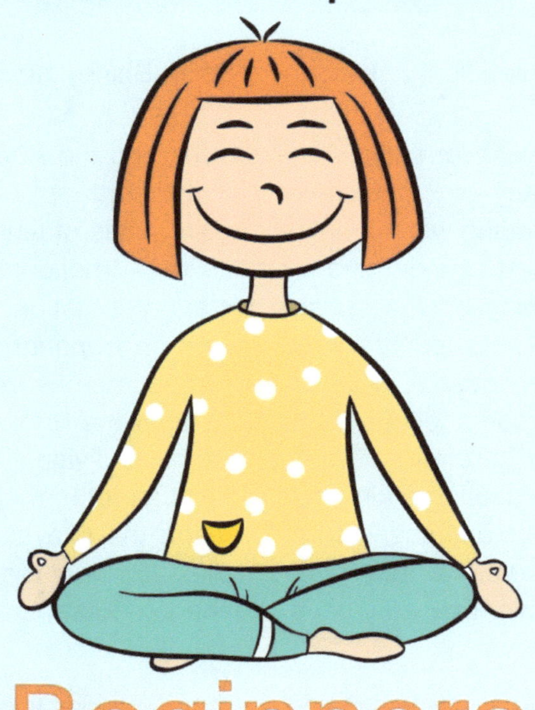

for Beginners

Eve Heidi Bine-Stock

Yana Bolbot

Contact the Author:
Eve Heidi Bine-Stock
P.O. Box 3346
Omaha, NE 68103
EveHeidiWrites@gmail.com

With love and thanks to my mother, Shirley Smalheiser.

Contents

Introduction

This book is for beginners. It is meant to be used beside your yoga mat, as a visual guide to poses and sequences. The most important information is provided right there, with each picture. No scrolling needed, no flipping pages back and forth for instructions.

For each main pose, this book shows you in pictures the preparatory and follow-up poses. No need to hunt through wordy descriptions to find this information (as other books require).

The charming illustrations in this book are meant to delight you and keep you motivated.

Don't worry if you can't do the poses "perfectly." You may not be able to touch your toes, or keep your legs straight during some poses. This will come with time and practice.

The benefits of practicing yoga are many. In addition to increased flexibility and strength, you can develop a calm and balance that overflows to other areas of your life.

Jump Right In!
A 10-Minute Beginner Sequence

Even though this is considered an "easy" sequence, you might not be able to do it every day when you first start. If needed, rest a day or two between sessions, and work your way down to shorter rest periods, until you *can* do it every day. Above all, listen to your body!

Here are some other guidelines:

- Do yoga on an empty stomach, so wait 1-2 hours after eating.

- Use an exercise mat. Practice in bare feet.

- Keep a pillow handy to use where indicated.

- Move slowly.

- Breathe in and out through your nose, if possible.

- Breathe slowly, deeply, and calmly during each pose. If you have trouble doing this, ease up on the pose until you can. No need to strain.

- Be mindful. Focus on what you are doing, and how your body feels, not on chores waiting for you.

Turn the page, and let's get started!

1.

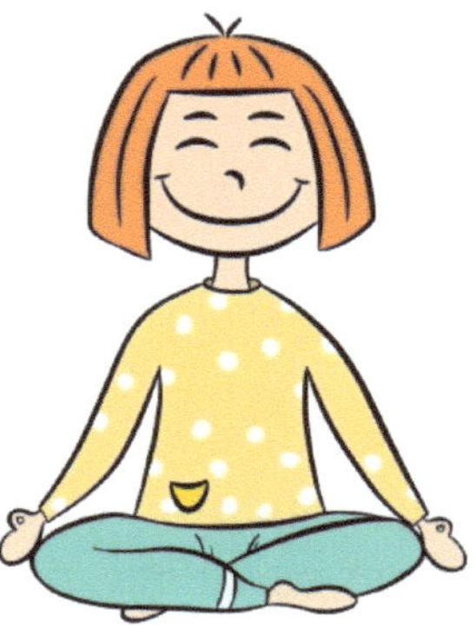

Easy Pose

If needed, sit on a pillow.
Cross legs at ankles.
Hold pose about 1 minute.
Next time you do sequence, reverse legs.

2.

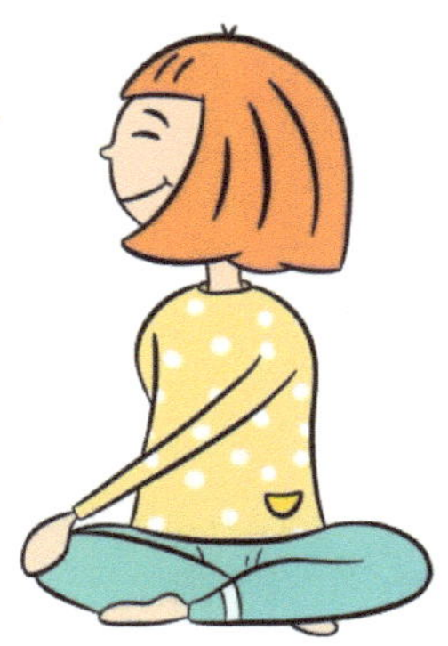

Seated Twist Pose

If needed, stay on pillow.
Twist right first & hold pose 6-8 breaths.
Repeat other side.

3.

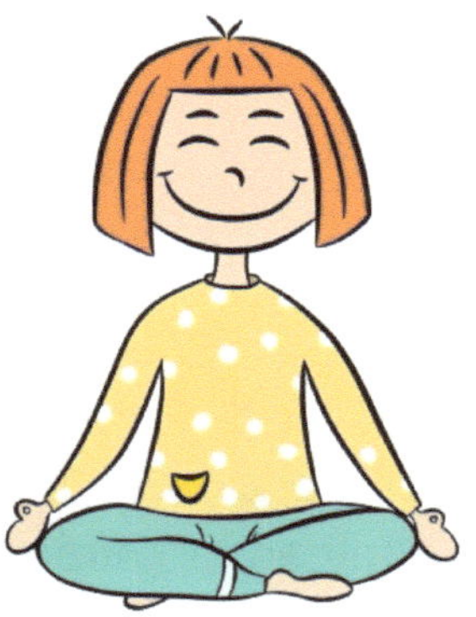

Easy Pose

If needed, stay on pillow.
Hold pose 2-3 breaths.

4.

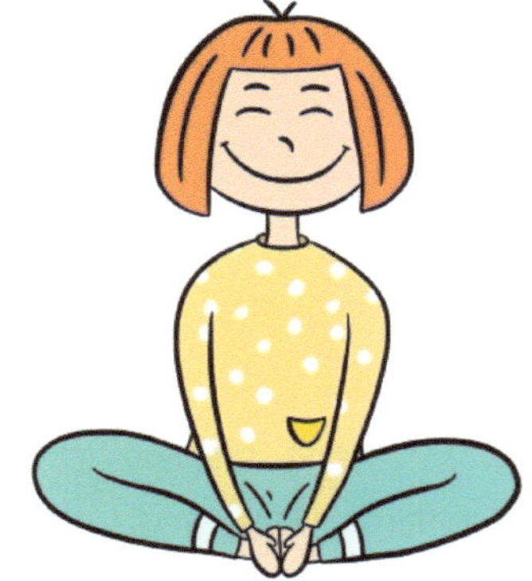

Butterfly Pose

Also called Bound Angle Pose.
Put soles of feet together.
If needed, stay on pillow.
Hold pose 6-8 breaths.

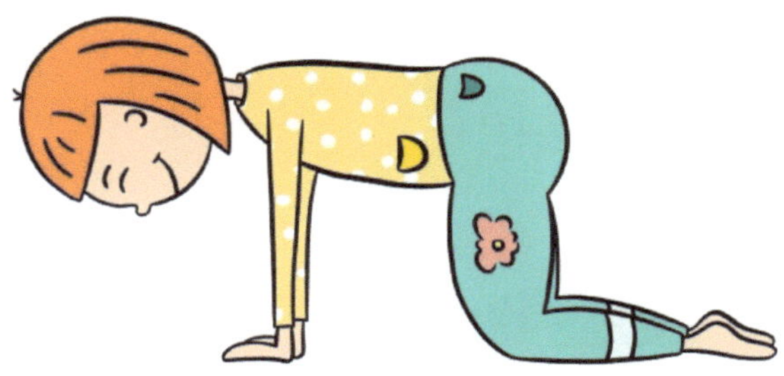

Table Top Pose

Also called Box Pose.
If needed, put pillow under knees.
Hold pose 2-3 breaths.

6.   7.

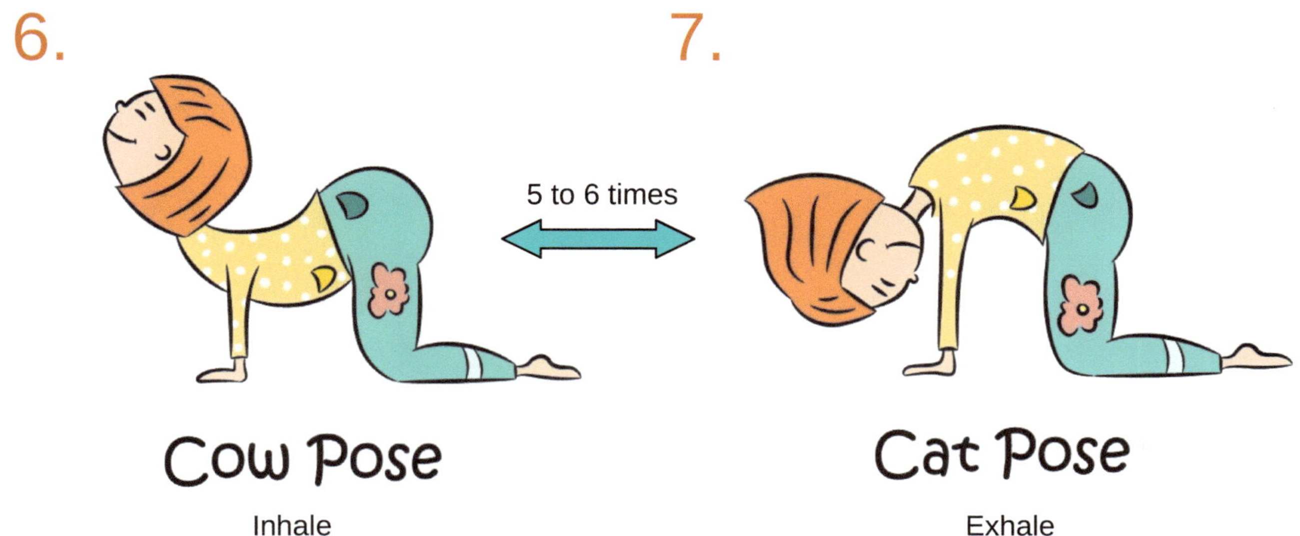

Cow Pose

Inhale

Cat Pose

Exhale

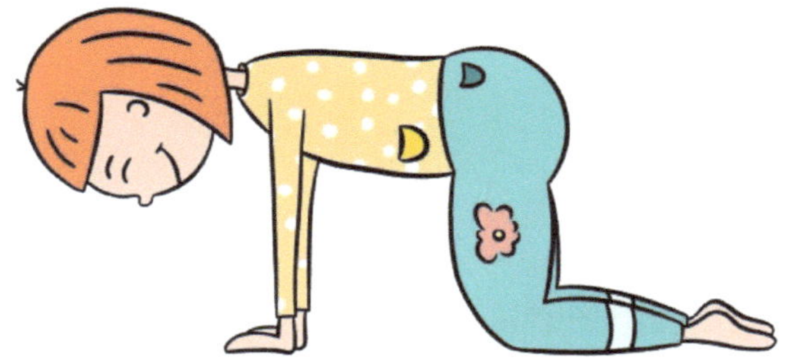

8.

Table Top Pose

Hold pose 2-3 breaths.

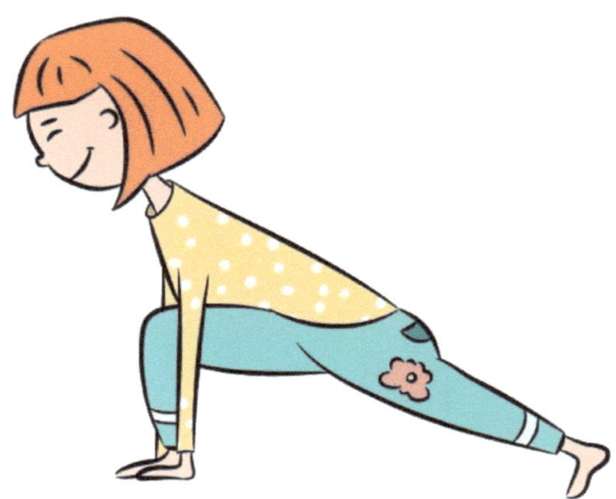

9.

Lunge Pose

Right leg first. Keep knee over ankle.
If needed, put back knee on floor,
with or without pillow.
Hold pose 6-8 breaths.
Repeat pose 8, then lunge with left leg.

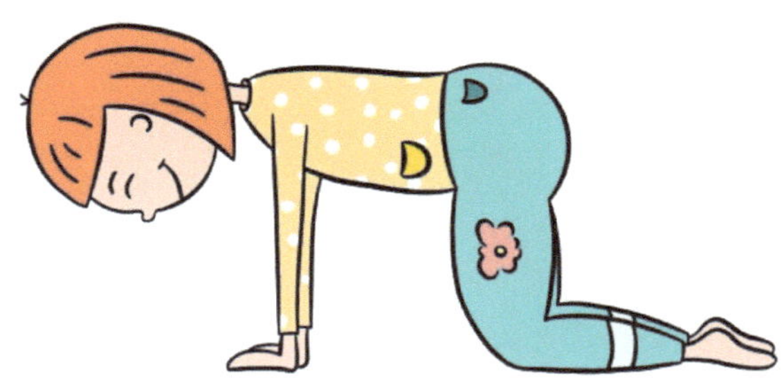

10.

Table Top Pose

Hold pose 2-3 breaths.

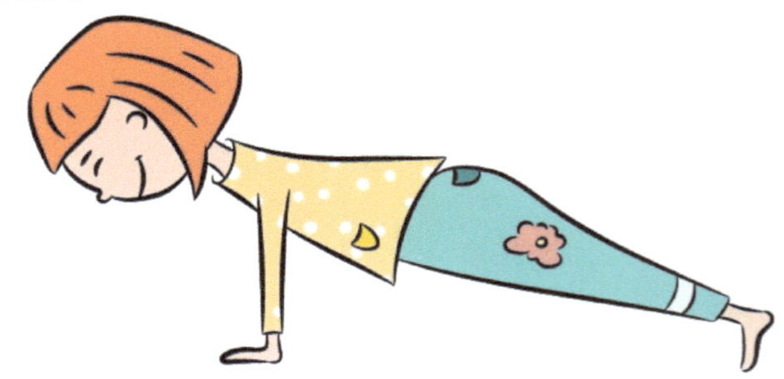

11.

Plank Pose

If needed, put knees on floor,
with or without pillow.
Hold pose 6-8 breaths.

12.

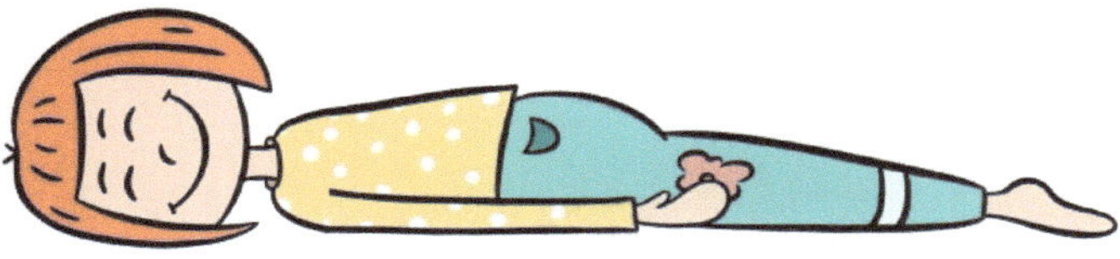

Front Corpse Pose

If needed, put pillow under
chest and pelvis.
Hold pose 5-6 breaths.

13.

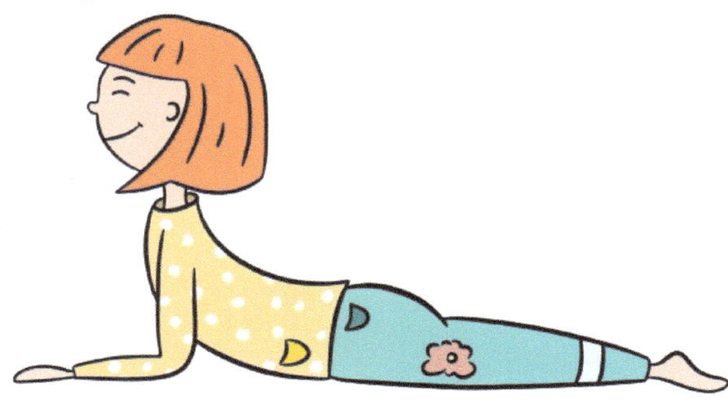

Sphinx Pose

Put forearms on floor, palms down.
Lift crown of head.
Hold pose 6-8 breaths.

14.

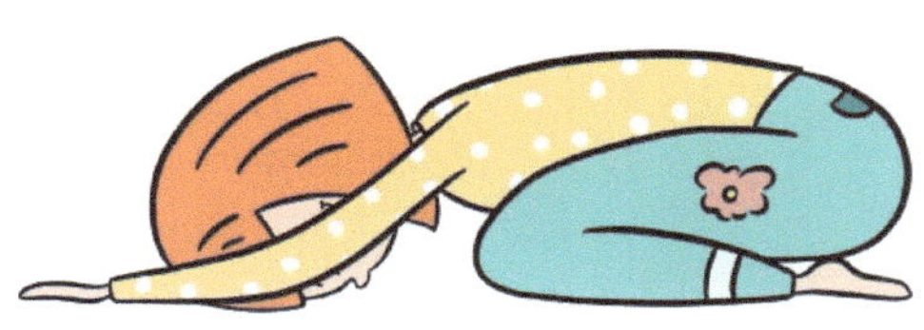

Extended
Child's Pose

Exhale as you fold.
If needed, put pillow under knees.
Hold pose 6-8 breaths.

15.

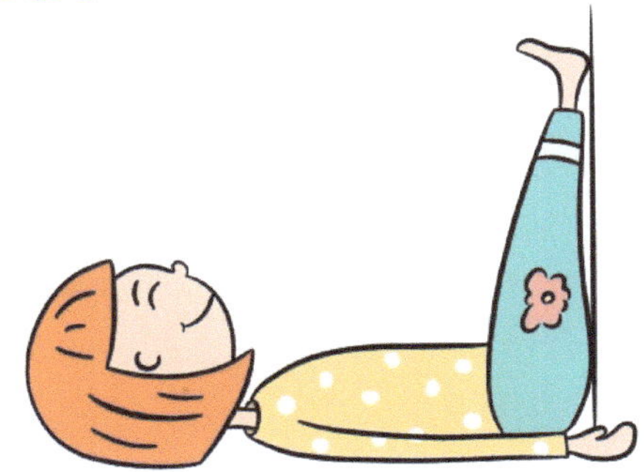

Legs Up the Wall Pose

Lean straight legs on a wall.
Hold pose 2-3 minutes.
Turn page for one more pose...

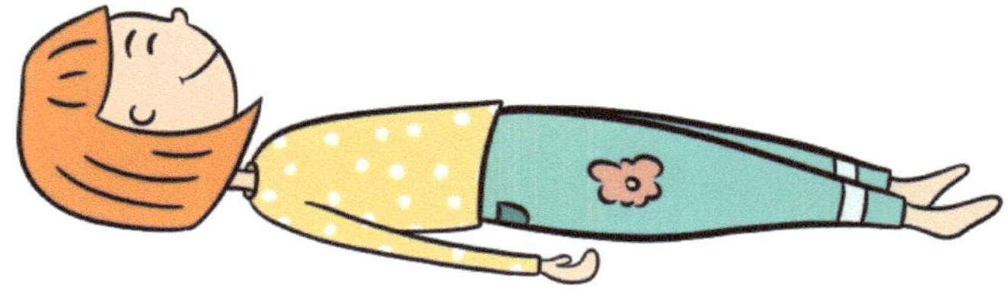

Corpse Pose

Also called Savasana.
Let feet and arms flop open.
If needed, put pillow under knees.
Hold pose 2-3 minutes.

Keep At It!
A 20-Minute Beginner Sequence

1. 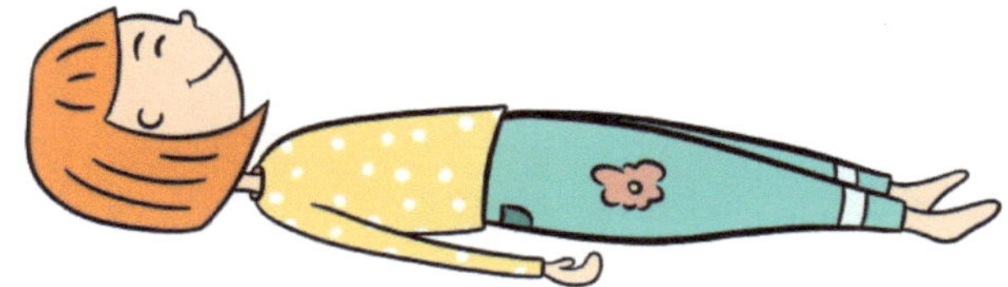

Corpse Pose

Also called Savasana.
Let feet and arms flop open.
If needed, put pillow under knees.
Hold pose 8-10 breaths.

3.

6 to 8 times

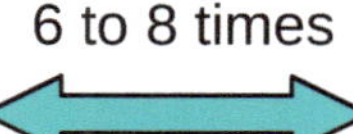

2. 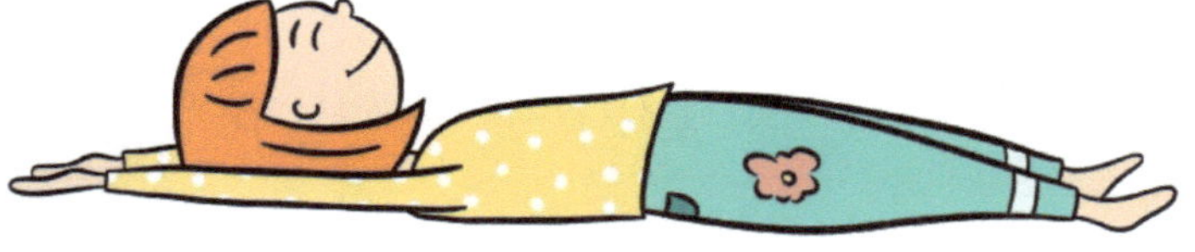

Extended Corpse Pose

Inhale as you raise arms.

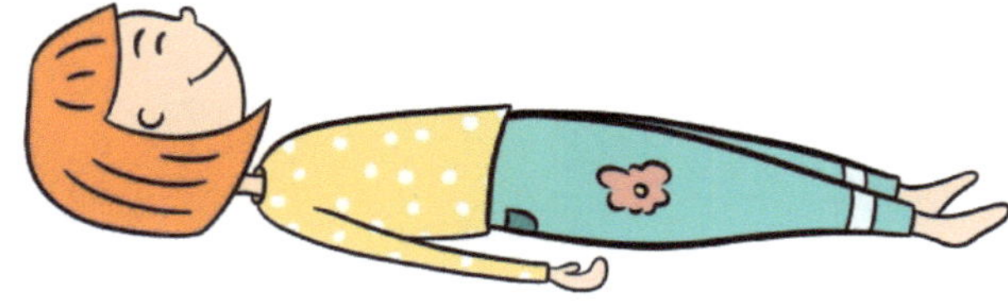

Corpse Pose

Exhale as you lower arms.

4.

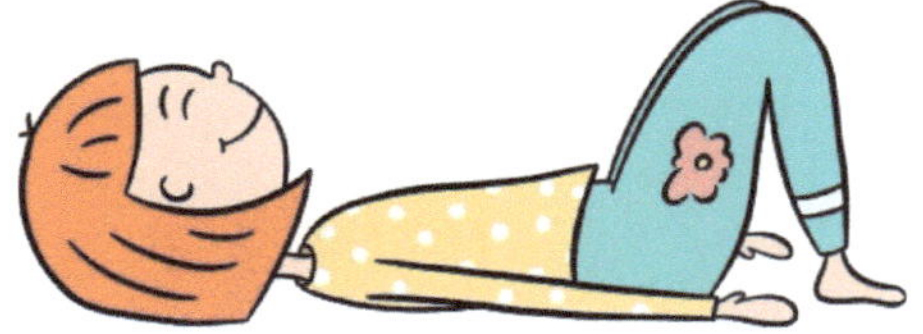

Preparation for Knee-to-Chest Pose

Hold pose 2-3 breaths.

5.

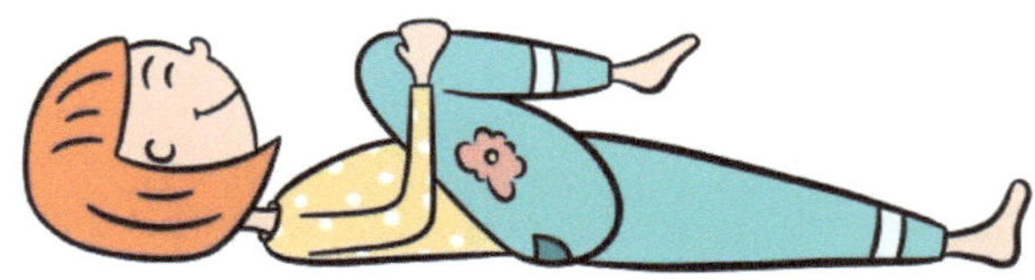

Knee-to-Chest Pose

Exhale as you lift right leg.
Grasp shin or thigh of right leg.
Hold pose 6-8 breaths.
Repeat pose 4, then lift left leg.

6.

7.

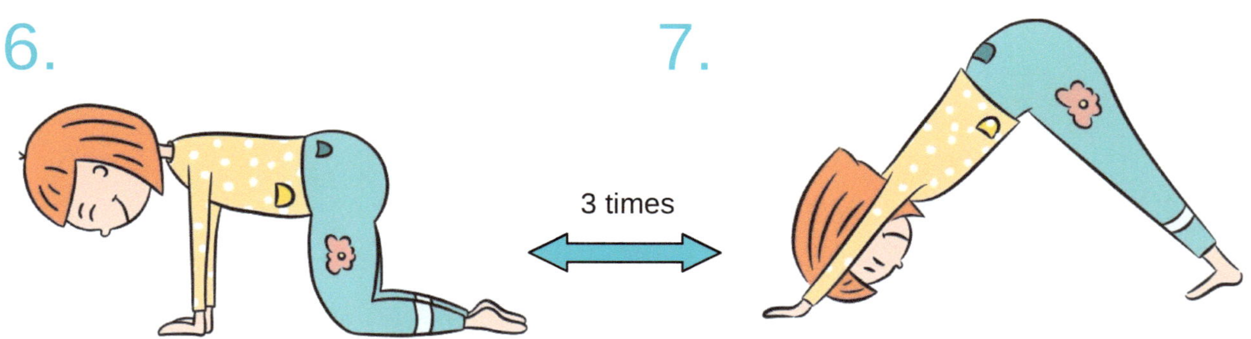

Table Top Pose

Inhale

Downward Facing Dog

Exhale as you lift hips and bend.
If needed, bend knees.
Repeat poses 6-7, 3 times,
then hold pose 7 for 6-8 breaths.

8.

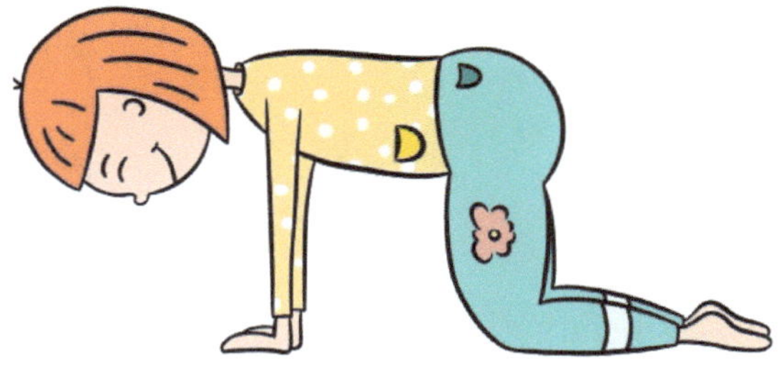

Table Top Pose

Hold pose 2-3 breaths.

9A.

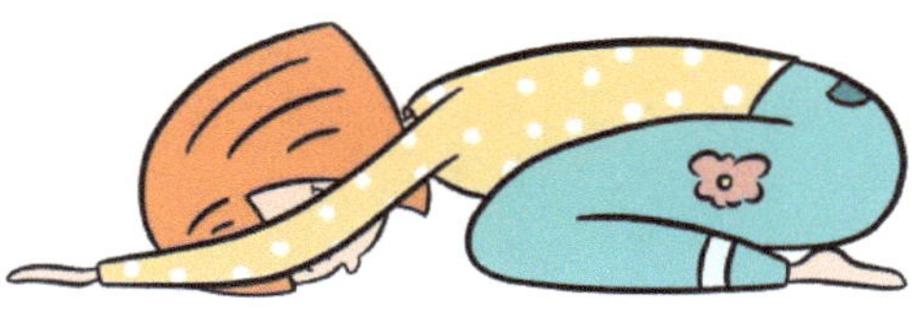

Extended
Child's Pose

Exhale as you fold.
If needed, put pillow under knees.
Hold pose 6-8 breaths.

OR

9B.

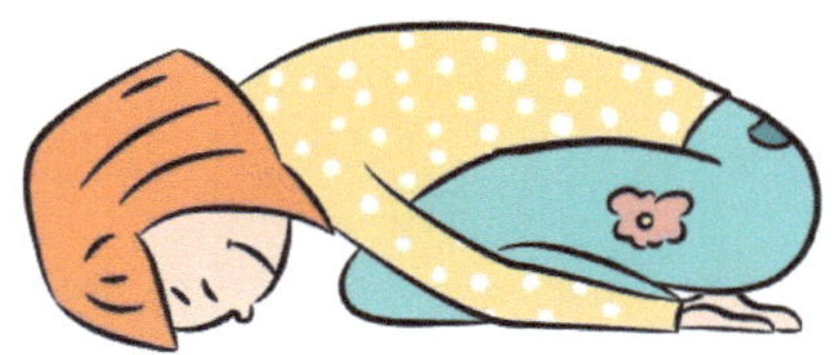

Child's Pose

Exhale as you fold.
If needed, put pillow under knees.
Hold pose 6-8 breaths.

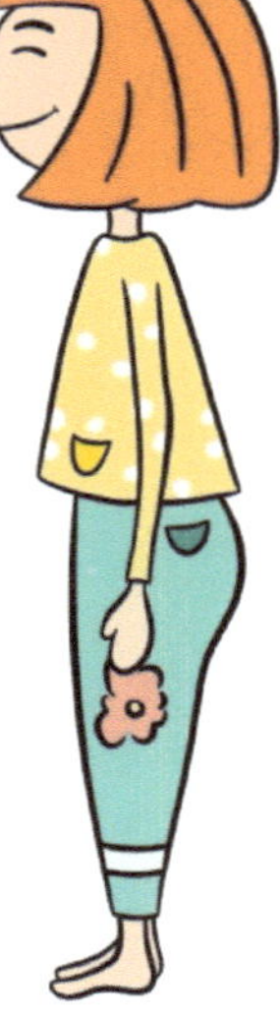

10.

Stack ankles, knees,
hips, & shoulders.
Lift crown of head.
Hold pose 2-3 breaths.

Mountain Pose

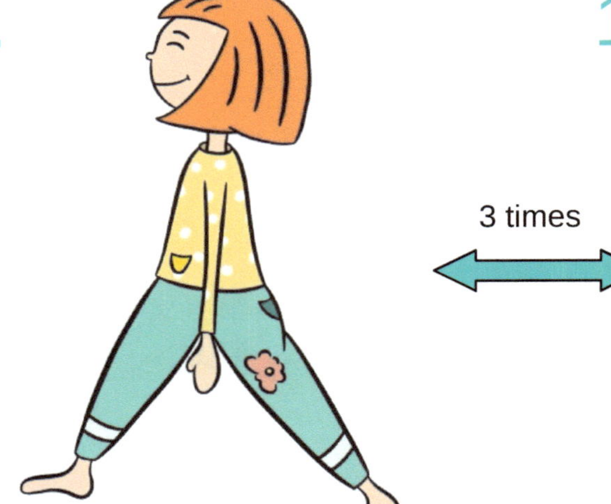

11.

Preparation for Crescent Pose

Exhale as you step right foot forward.

3 times

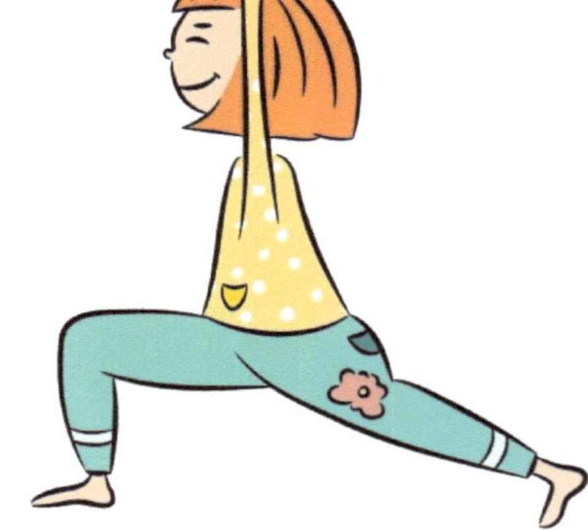

12.

Crescent Pose

Inhale as you raise arms & bend right leg.
Keep front knee directy above ankle.
Repeat poses 11 & 12, 3 times,
then hold pose 12 for 6-8 breaths.
Repeat poses 10-12 with left leg.

13.

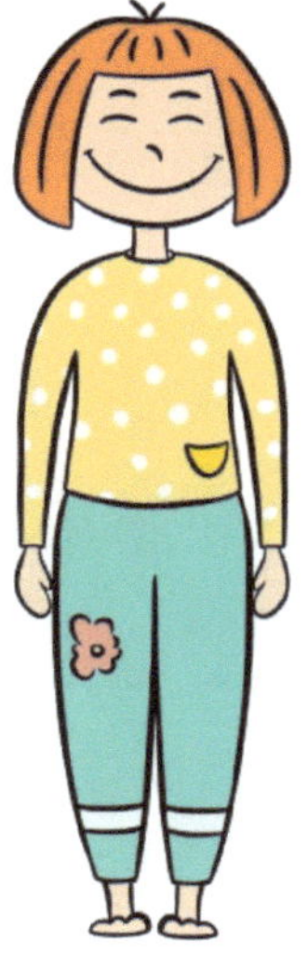

Mountain Pose

Inhale & exhale.

14.

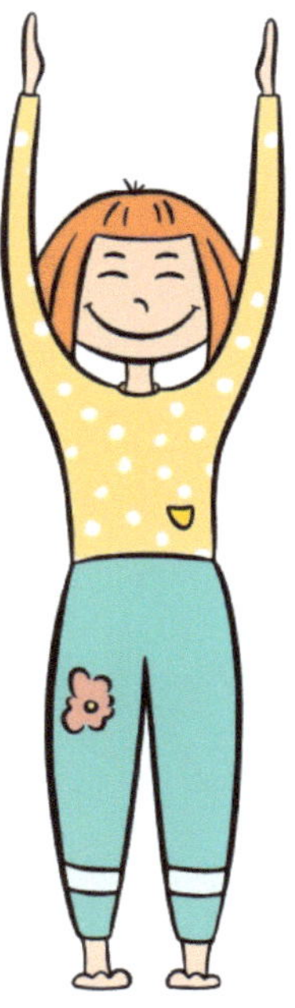

Extended
Mountain Pose

Inhale as you raise arms.

15.

Roll your back up
(stacking vertebrae)
until back is straight.
Inhale as you roll up.

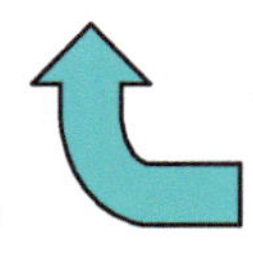

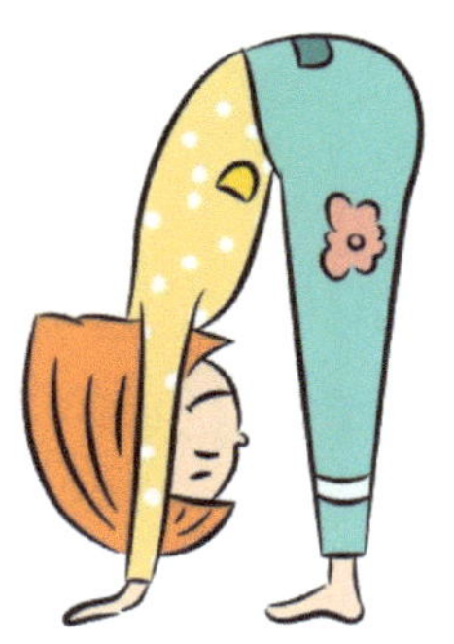

Exhale as you bend forward.
If needed, bend knees.
Repeat poses 13-15, 3 times,
then hold pose 15 for 6-8 breaths.

Standing Forward
Bend Pose

16.

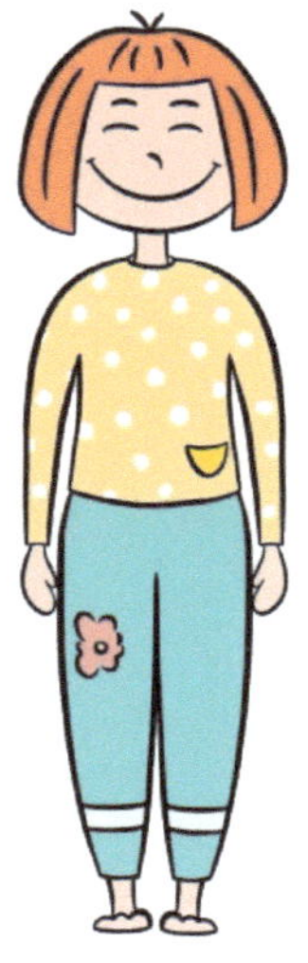

Mountain Pose

Hold pose 2-3 breaths.

17.

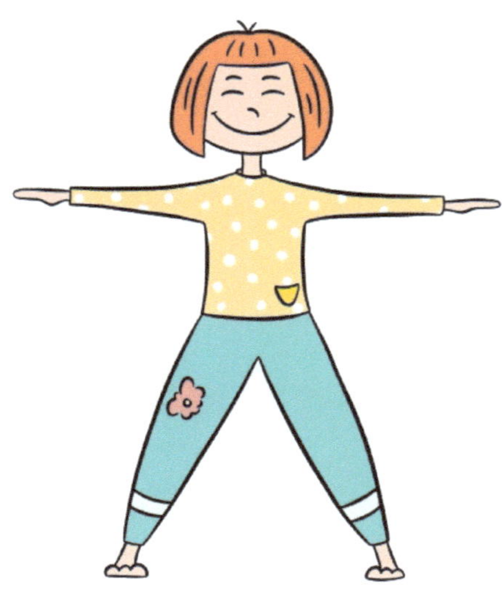

Five-Pointed Star Pose

Inhale as you take pose.
Hold pose 2-3 breaths.

18.

Standing Wide-Legged Forward Bend

Exhale as you bend forward.
If needed, bend knees.
Hold pose 6-8 breaths.
Just go as far down as you can.
Don't strain.

19.

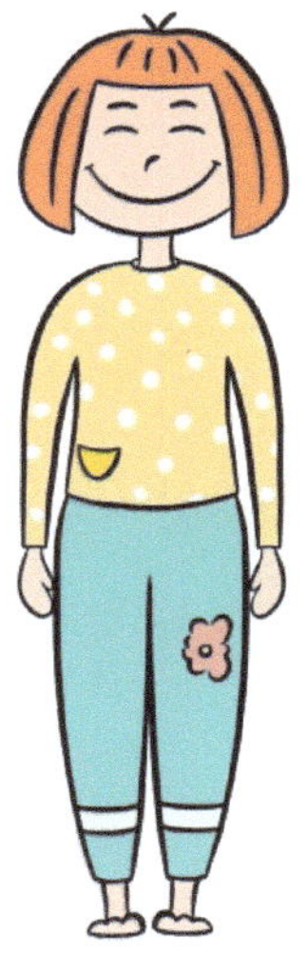

Mountain Pose

Hold pose 2-3 breaths.

20.

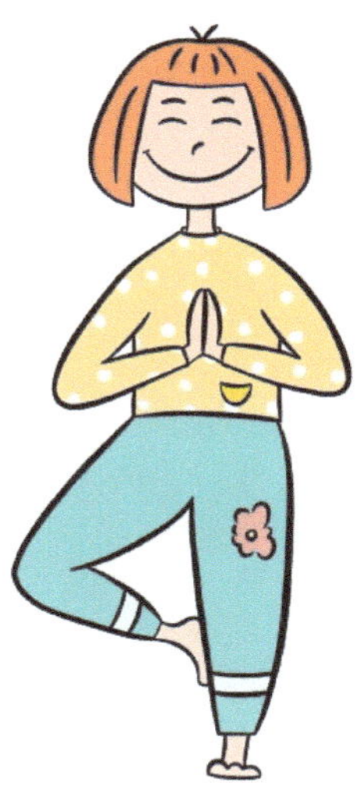

Tree Pose

Shift weight to left leg.
Exhale and lift & bend right leg.
Note: foot should be above or below
the knee,not on it.
Hold pose 6-8 breaths.
Repeat pose 19, then shift weight to
right leg, and lift & bend left leg.

21.

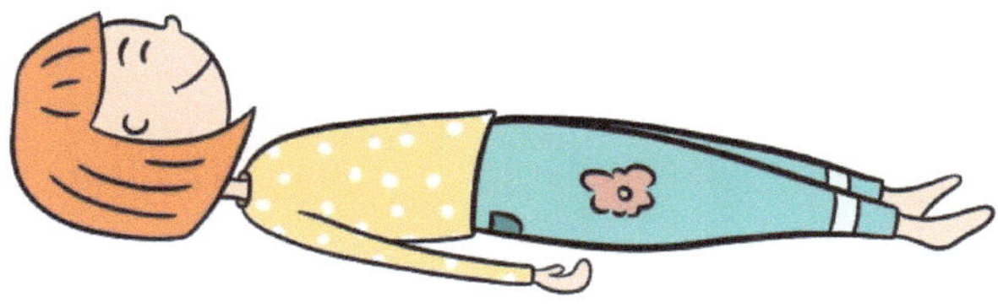

Corpse Pose

Also called Savasana.
Let feet and arms flop open.
If needed, put pillow under knees.
Hold pose 2-3 minutes.

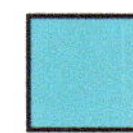

Go with the Flow
Sun Salutation

Sun Salutation (also called Surya Namaskar or Surya Namaskara) is a sequence of 12 poses performed in a smooth, graceful flow.

The breath is a very important part of this sequence. Moving from one pose to the next is always done as you either inhale or exhale. The diagram shows you which breath—inhalation or exhalation—to take as you enter a pose.

You can control the pace of the sequence by changing the number of breaths you take in each pose. Just be sure that you move to the next pose with the right breath.

Do one complete Sun Salutation with your right leg forward for the Lunge in steps 4 & 8, then do a second complete Sun Salutation with your left leg forward for the Lunge.

There are many variations available for the Sun Salutation; I have shown you one for beginners.

Before getting to the sequence itself, get to know four poses on the next page that have not yet been introduced, but appear in this Sun Salutation sequence.

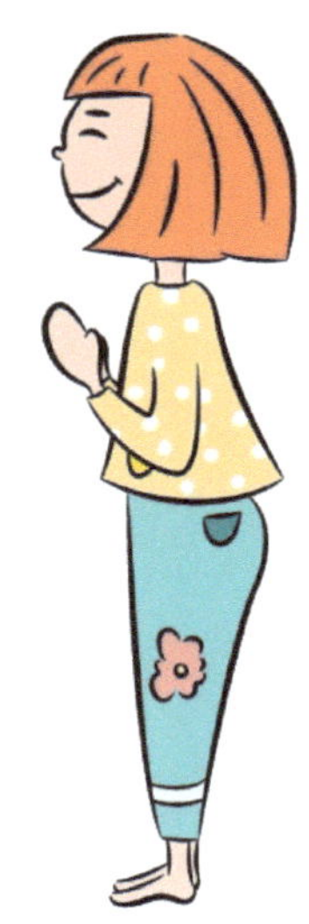

Prayer Pose

Similar to Mountain, but with
hands held in a praying gesture.

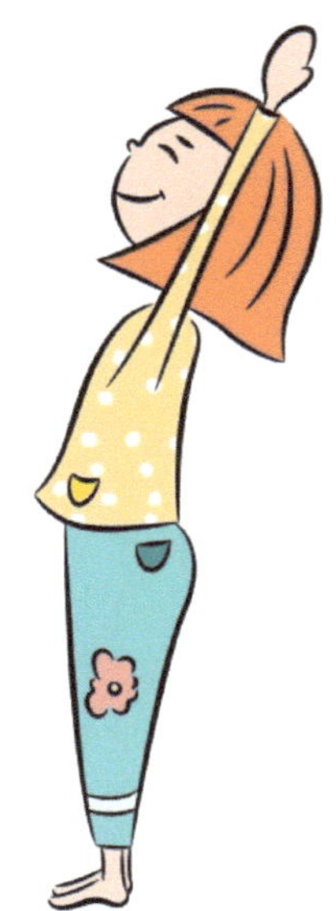

Raised Hands Pose

Similar to Extended Mountain,
but with a gentle backbend.

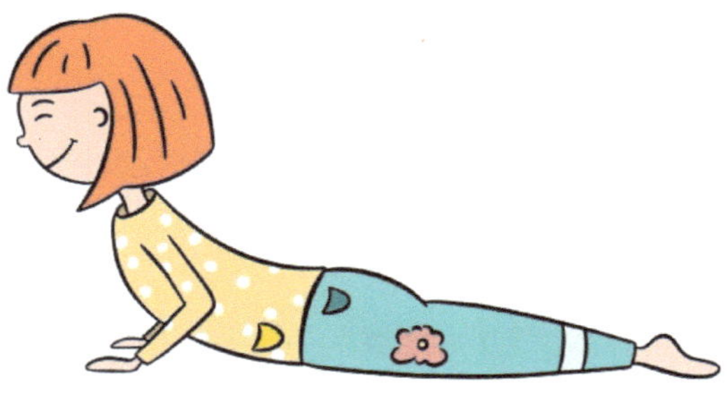

Low Cobra

Also called Baby Cobra.
Similar to Sphinx, but with
palms, not forearms, on mat.

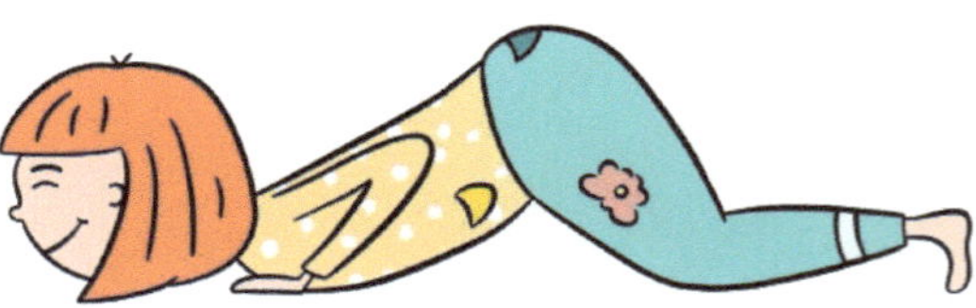

Knees-Chest-Chin Pose

Also called Eight Point Pose.
Touch floor with toes, knees,
hands, chest, & chin.

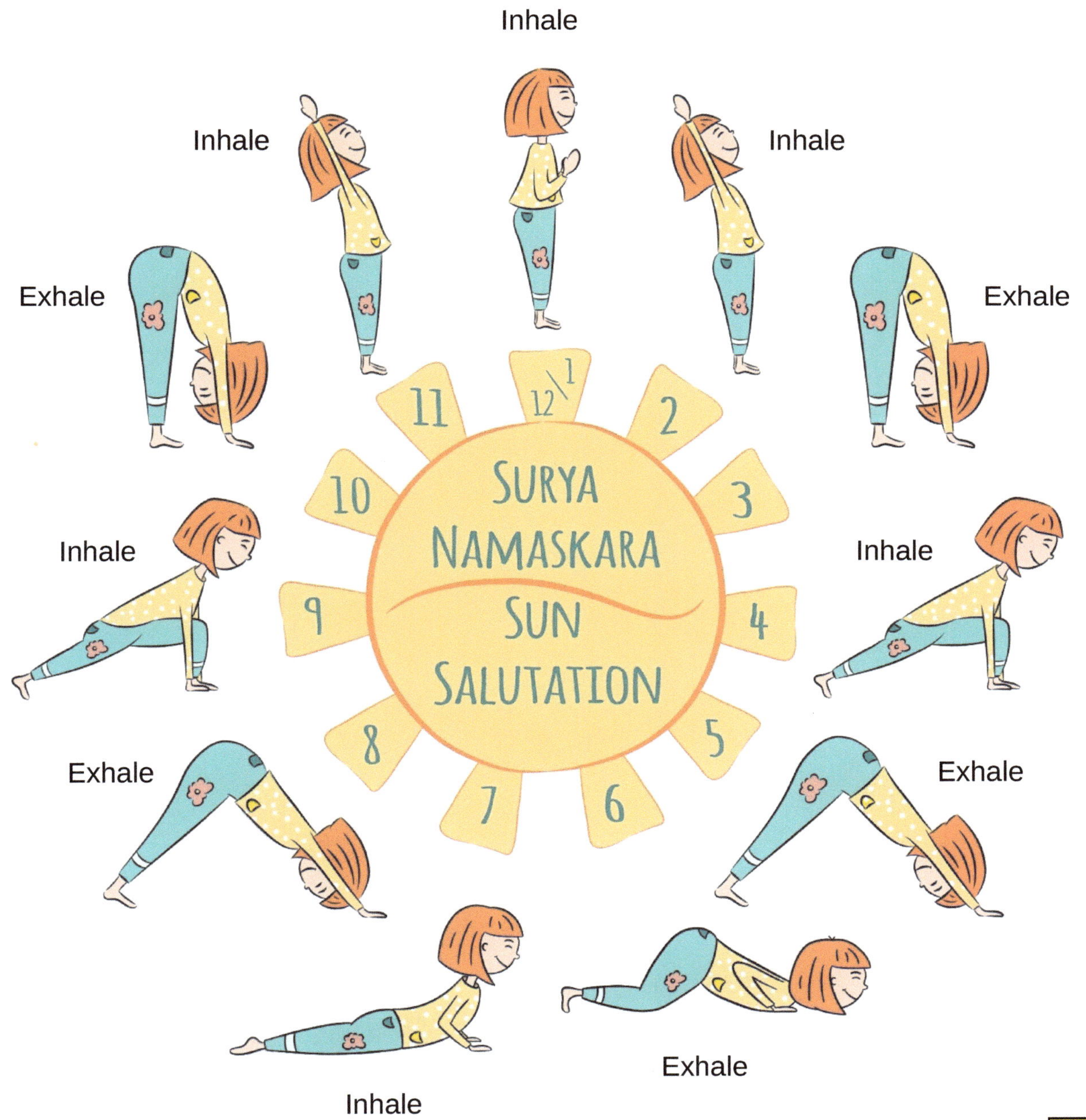

Inhale
Inhale
Inhale
Exhale
Exhale
11
12 1
2
10
3
SURYA
NAMASKARA
SUN
SALUTATION
9
4
Inhale
Inhale
8
5
Exhale
7 6
Exhale
Exhale
Inhale

Mix it Up!

Other Essential Beginner Poses

1. Chair Pose

Preparatory Pose: Extended Mountain Pose 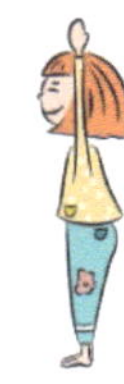

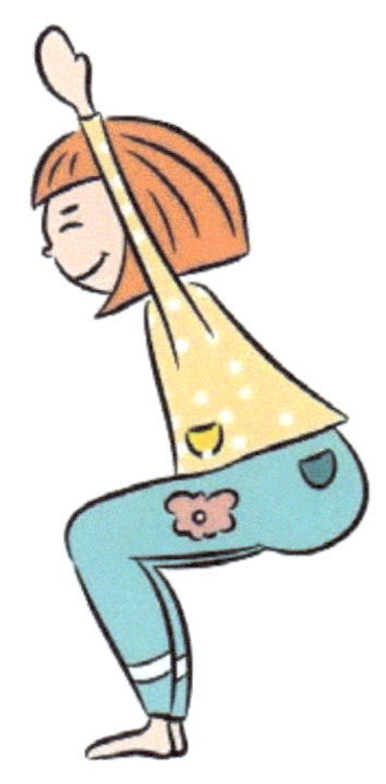

Chair Pose

Exhale as you bend knees and "sit."
Hold pose 5-6 breaths.

Follow-up Pose: Standing Forward Bend 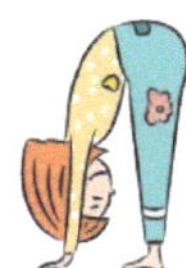

2. Warrior 1 Pose

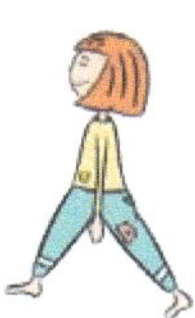

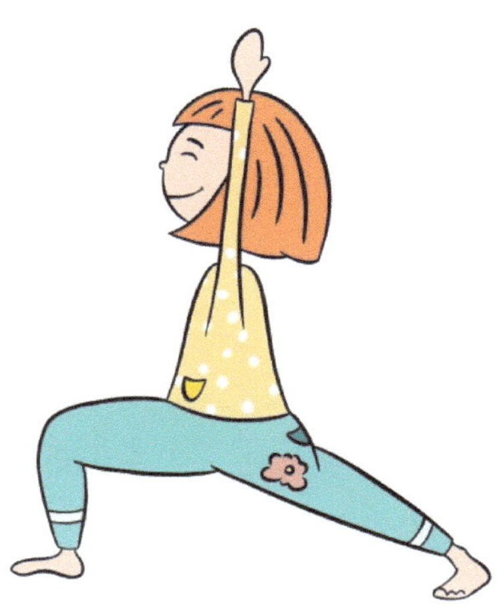

Warrior 1 Pose

From Preparatory Pose, turn back foot so its arch lines up with front heel.
Inhale as you bend knee, turn hips to face front, and lift arms above head.
Keep front knee directy above ankle.
Hold pose 6-8 breaths.
Repeat with other leg.

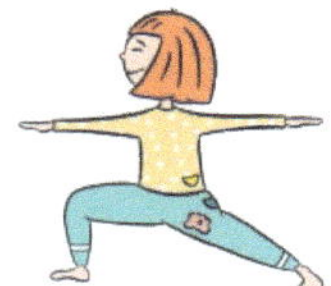

3. Warrior 2 Pose

 Prep to Warrior 2 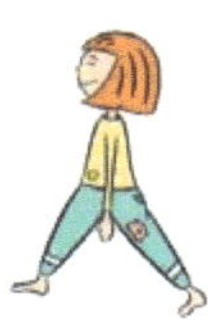

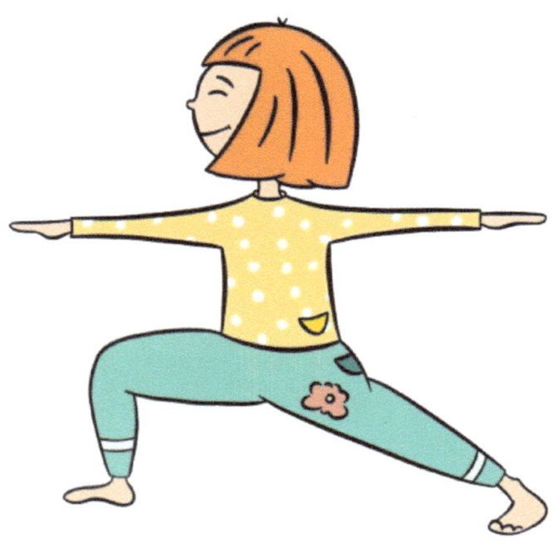

Warrior 2 Pose

From Preparatory Pose, turn back foot so its arch lines up with front heel.
Inhale as you bend knee, turn hips out, and lift arms to form a T.
Keep head facing toward fingertips.
Keep front knee directy above ankle.
Hold pose 6-8 breaths.
Repeat with other leg.

Follow-up Pose: Side Angle 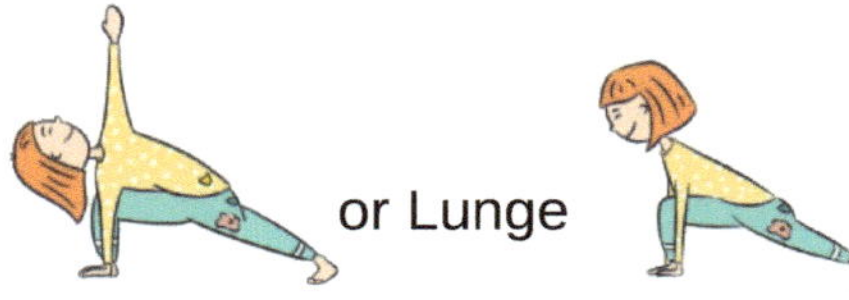 or Lunge

4. Side Angle Pose

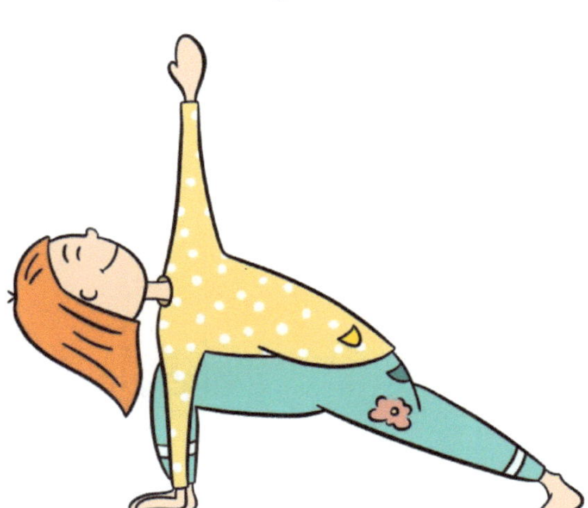

Side Angle Pose

From Warrior 2 Pose, exhale as you bend to the side.
Keep front knee directy above ankle.
If needed, rest forearm on thigh of bent leg.
Hold pose 6-8 breaths.
Repeat other side.

Follow-up Pose: Warrior 2

5. Staff Pose

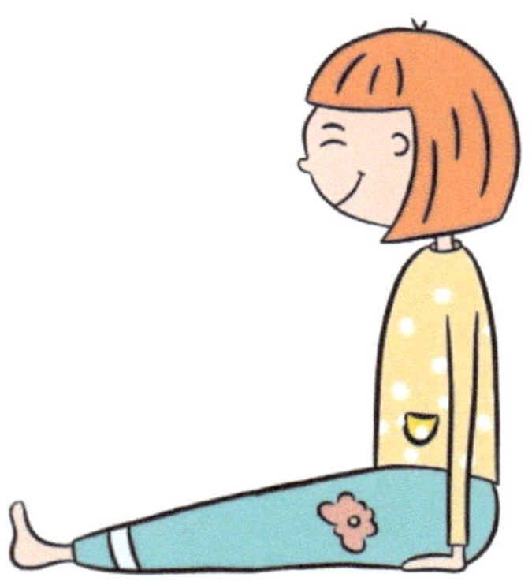

Staff Pose

If needed, sit on pillow.
Press palms on floor. Press thighs & heels down.
Keep knees & heels together. Flex feet & spread toes.
Draw abdomen in toward spine. Keep spine long & straight.
Stack hips & shoulders. Lift crown of head.
Hold pose 6-8 breaths.

Follow-up Pose: Downward Facing Dog 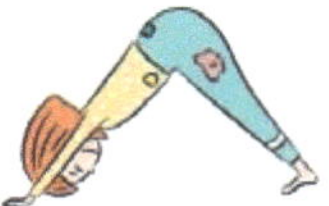 or Standing Forward Bend

6. Low Boat Pose

Preparatory Pose: Staff Pose 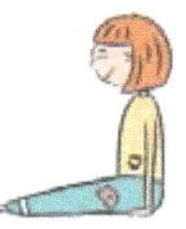 or Corpse Pose 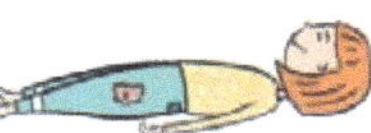

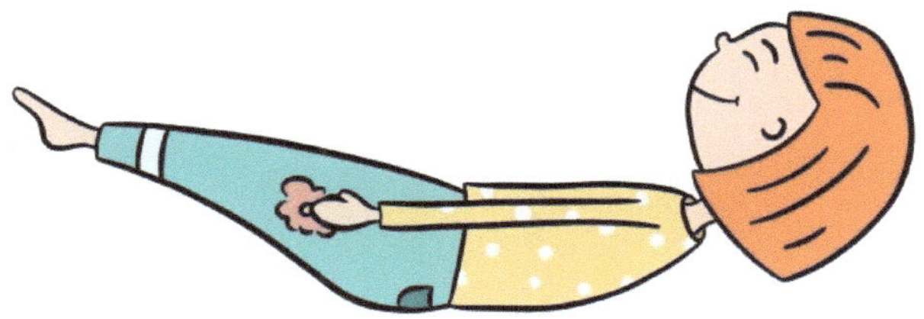

Low Boat Pose

From Staff Pose, lower your torso & shoulders,
and lift legs, keeping them straight.
From Corpse Pose, Inhale as you lift your head,
shoulders, torso, arms and legs.
Feet & head should hover about six inches above floor.
Hold pose 6-8 breaths.

Follow-up Pose: Corpse Pose

7. Garland Pose

Preparatory Pose: Prayer Pose 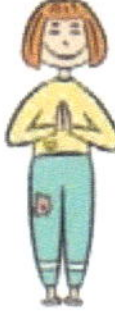

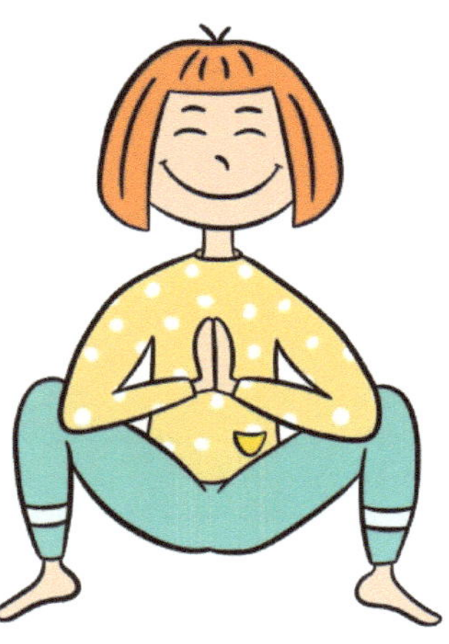

Garland Pose

From Prayer Pose, step feet about mat's width apart.
Exhale as you lower hips & bend knees, into a squat.
If heels don't touch floor, support them with folded towel.
Hold for 5-6 breaths.
To release, put fingertips on floor,
and slowly straighten legs, moving into follow-up pose.

Follow-up Pose: Downward Facing Dog 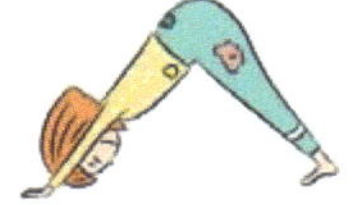 or Standing Forward Bend 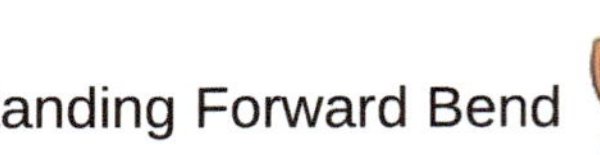

8. Thunderbolt Pose

Preparatory Pose: Table Top Pose 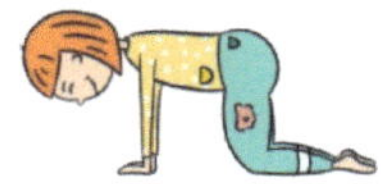

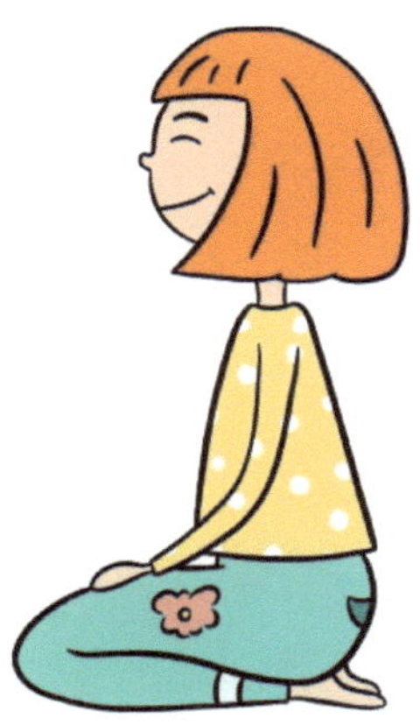

Thunderbolt Pose

Exhale and sit on heels.
If needed, put pillow between calves & thighs.
Try to hold pose for 1 minute.

Follow-up Pose: Table Top Pose 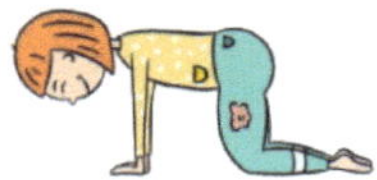

9. Hero Pose

Preparatory Pose: Table Top Pose 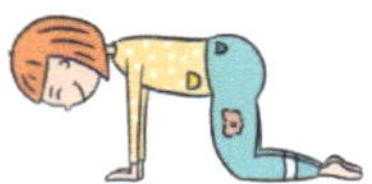

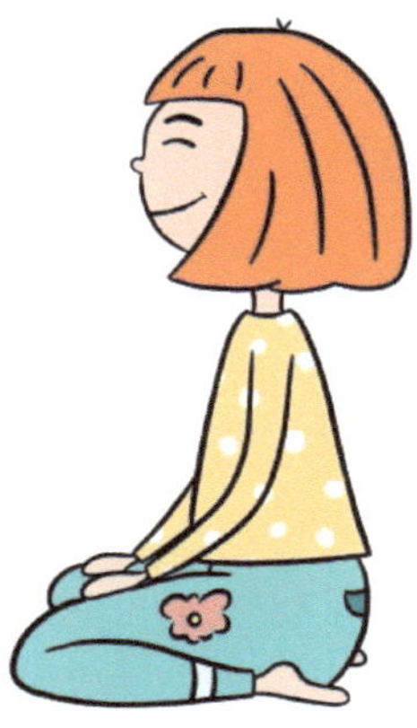

Hero Pose

Exhale and sit on mat between feet.
If needed, sit on book(s) placed between feet.
Try to hold pose for 1 minute.

Follow-up Pose: Table Top Pose 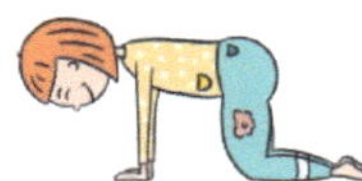

10. Happy Baby Pose

 Corpse Pose 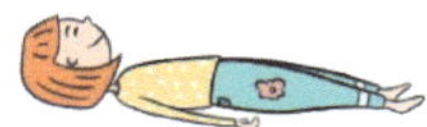

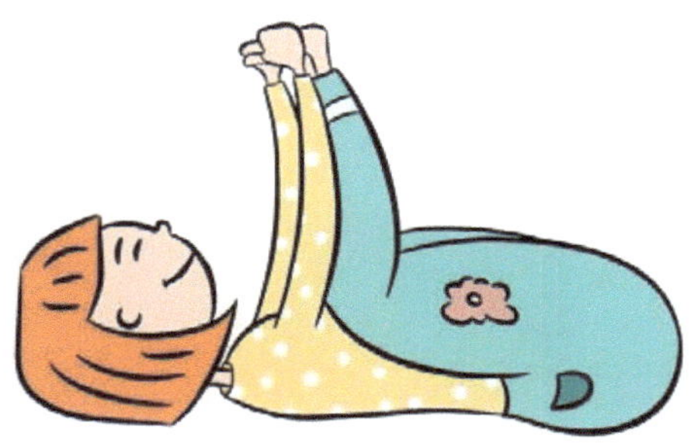

Happy Baby Pose

From Corpse Pose, bring knees to chest.
Spread feet & knees wide, while grasping outside of feet.
If your neck lifts off mat, grasp ankles or shins, instead.
If desired, rock gently from side to side.
Hold pose 8-12 breaths.

Follow-up Pose: Corpse Pose 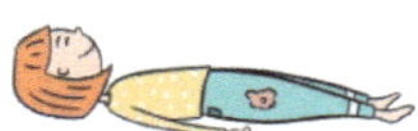

11. Bow Pose

 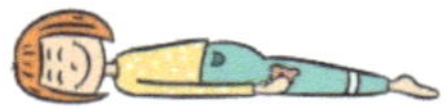

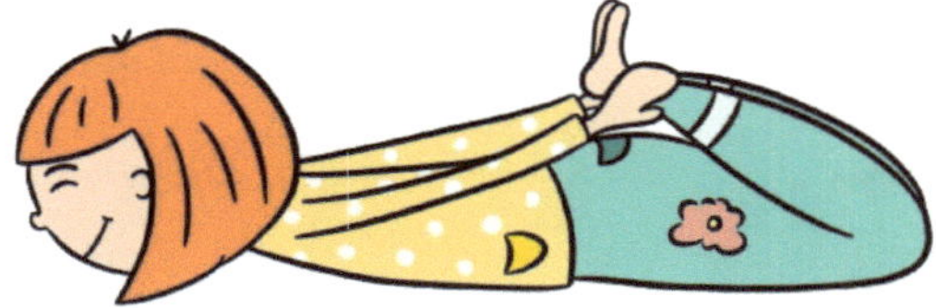

Preparation for Bow Pose

From Front Corpse, exhale & bend knees.
Grasp ankles.
If needed, put pillow under hips.

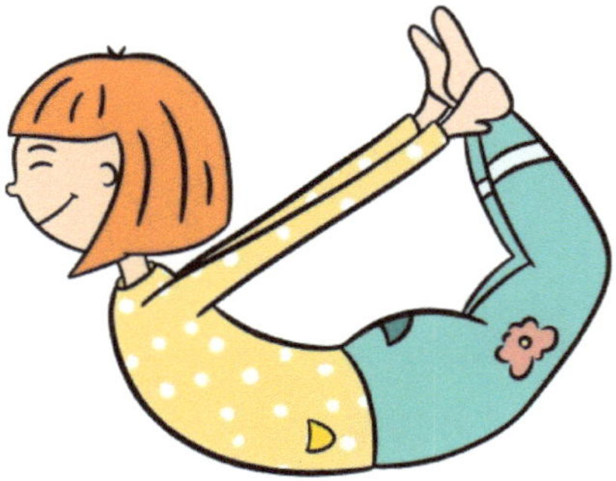

Bow Pose

Inhale & lift feet, thighs, head & chest.
Hold pose 5-6 breaths.

.

Follow-up Pose: Front Corpse Pose 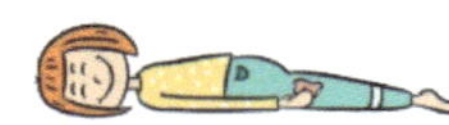

12. Forearm Plank Pose

Preparatory Pose: Sphinx Pose 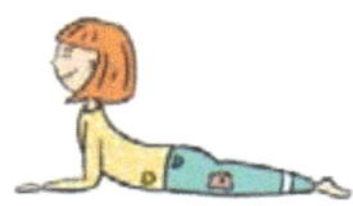

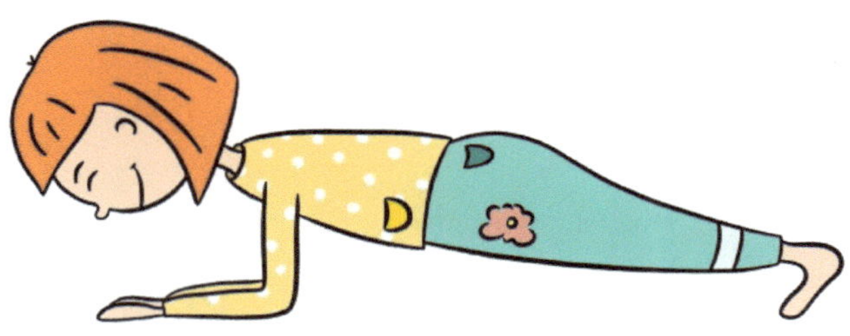

Forearm Plank Pose

From Sphinx Pose, lift belly first, then hips, then thighs, then knees.
Hold pose 5-6 breaths.
To come down, lower your body in reverse order,
then move into follow-up pose.

Follow-up Pose: Extended Child's Pose 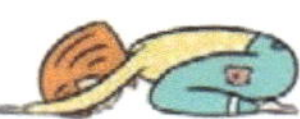

What's Next?
Additional Resources

I recommend the following Web site to learn more about yoga for beginners:

www.YogaBasics.com

This Web site has photographs; clear and straightforward instructions; modifications; contraindications; and preparatory and follow-up poses.

Here are three seasoned yoga teachers who are non-judgmental and non-snobby. They are yoga teachers for real people. Their videos are available online, as shown below: They will take you to the next level.

Adriene Mishler
Search YouTube.com for Yoga with Adriene

Erin Motz
Search YouTube.com for Bad Yogi

Christina D'Arrigo
Search YouTube.com for Chriska Yoga

Have fun, and best wishes for a satisfying yoga journey!